EMPOWERING THE CHILD WITH INTELLECTUAL DISABILITY

A GUIDE FOR PARENTS AND FAMILIES

Dr. A. MITRA, MBBS, MD, DMI.

Disclaimer:

The information provided in this book, "Empowering the Child with Intellectual Disability," is intended for educational purposes only. While every effort has been made to ensure accuracy and relevance, readers are advised to consult healthcare professionals for personalized advice and treatment options tailored to individual circumstances. The author and publisher disclaim any liability arising directly or indirectly from the use or application of the contents of this book.

DEDICATION

This is a tribute to the heroes in parents and families who, with their ceaseless love, resilience, and commitment, provide children with Intellectual Disability the strength to overcome obstacles and flourish. The steadfast bravery and perseverance of these families serve as an inspiration to us all.

EMPOWERING THE CHILD WITH INTELLECTUAL
DISABILITY

CONTENTS

- Therapists: Occupational therapists, speech-language pathologists, and physical therapists
- Social workers: Connecting families to resources and support services
- Working Together as a Team

- Understanding your child's rights and entitlements
- How to Find Out What Your Child Qualifies For
- Effective communication with educators and healthcare providers
- Helping Your Child Practice Speaking Up
- Growing Independence
- Building partnerships with schools and community organizations
- Finding People to Help
- Using Technology to Stay Connected

- Learning styles
- Effective teaching strategies
- Differentiated instruction
- Celebrating progress and growth
- Help people with ID keep growing

- Dealing with bullying and social exclusion
- Promoting social inclusion

- Prioritizing your own mental and physical well-being
- Finding support groups and connecting with other families
- Strategies for managing stress and avoiding burnout
- Maintaining healthy relationships
- Prioritizing relaxation and stress-reduction techniques
- Respite care services
- Seeking professional help

- Fostering understanding and empathy among siblings
- Encouraging shared activities and creating opportunities for connection
- Addressing sibling rivalry and jealousy
- Celebrating the unique bond between siblings of a Child with ID
- Addressing sibling guilt and resentment

- Encouraging sibling participation in caregiving
- Celebrating sibling differences
- Building a lifelong support system

- Understanding financial resources available to families with ID
- Government benefits and assistance programs
- Securing the Future
- Utilizing insurance coverage effectively

- Guardianship options
- Transition to adulthood
- Long-term care planning
- Addressing end-of-life decisions

- Importance of recognizing achievements
- Creating traditions and rituals to acknowledge achievements
- Setting realistic goals and celebrating progress along the way
- Finding joy in the journey

- Building a legacy of love and acceptance
- Resources

xii

ACKNOWLEDGMENTS

I extend heartfelt gratitude to all who contributed to "Empowering the Child with Intellectual Disability." Thanks to the courageous children and families for sharing their experiences. Deep appreciation to healthcare professionals, therapists, educators, and researchers for their dedication. Special thanks to colleagues, friends, and mentors for their unwavering support and feedback. Gratitude also to the publishing team for their hard work. This book is a testament to a compassionate community dedicated to empowering children with Intellectual Disability and fostering inclusivity.

Thank you all.

Dr. A. Mitra

1. UNDERSTANDING INTELLECTUAL DISABILITY

What is ID?

Intellectual disability (ID) means someone has a brain condition that affects how they learn and do everyday things. It starts before they are 22 years old and lasts their whole life. There are two main things to consider with ID:

- **Learning:** People with ID may have trouble learning new things or understanding information.
- **Daily Activities:** They might need some help with things like getting dressed, talking to others, or taking care of themselves.

Types of ID

There are different levels of ID, depending on how much help someone needs:

- **Mild ID:** This is most common. People with mild ID can often live on their own with some support and may have jobs.
- **Moderate ID:** People with moderate ID need more help with daily activities but can still learn some things.

- **Severe ID:** People with severe ID need a lot of help with daily activities and may have trouble communicating.
- **Profound ID:** This is the least common type. People with profound ID need a lot of help with everything and may have very limited communication skills.

What causes ID?

There are many reasons why someone might have ID. Sometimes it is because of a problem with their genes, like Down syndrome. Other times, it can happen before birth because of things like the mom being sick or not getting enough nutrients. Problems during birth or serious illnesses later in life can also cause ID. In many cases, doctors do not know the exact reason.

Medical Causes of Intellectual Disability

Here is a list of some common medical causes of Intellectual Disability (ID):

Genetic Conditions:
- Down syndrome
- Fragile X syndrome
- Prader-Willi syndrome
- Williams syndrome
- Angelman syndrome

- Tuberous sclerosis complex
- Phenylketonuria (PKU)
- Tay-Sachs disease

Chromosomal Abnormalities:
- Trisomy 13 (Patau syndrome)
- Trisomy 18 (Edwards syndrome)

Prenatal factors:
- Maternal infections (e.g., rubella, cytomegalovirus)
- Alcohol exposure during pregnancy
- Fetal alcohol syndrome (FAS)
- Drug exposure during pregnancy
- Premature birth
- Low birth weight

Perinatal factors:
- Oxygen deprivation at birth
- Infections during childbirth (e.g., meningitis)

Postnatal factors:
- Head trauma
- Severe childhood illnesses (e.g., meningitis, encephalitis)
- Lead poisoning
- Mercury poisoning

Metabolic Disorders:
- Phenylketonuria (PKU)
- Maple syrup urine disease
- Galactosemia

Note: This list is not exhaustive and it is important to consult with a healthcare professional for a diagnosis.

Important things to know:

- ID is not a disease; it is a lifelong condition.
- With help and support, people with ID can live happy and fulfilling lives.
- Everyone with ID is different and has their own strengths and challenges.

Going Through an Intellectual Disability (ID) Assessment

What is an ID Assessment?

An ID assessment is a series of tests and meetings to see if someone has Intellectual Disability (ID). The assessment helps figure out the best ways to support the person.

Who is Involved?

A team of doctors and specialists usually do the assessment. This might include a psychologist, teacher, or therapist. The tests can be done at a clinic, hospital, or even a school.

What Happens During the Assessment?

There are a few things the team will do:

- **Talk to you:** They will ask questions about the person's health and development since they were born.
- **Do Tests:** These tests see how well the person can learn and do things on their own.
- **Observe the Person:** The team will watch how the person interacts with others and does things.
- **Maybe More Tests:** Sometimes, the doctor might order blood tests or other tests to see if there is another reason for the challenges.

Getting Ready for the Assessment

Here are some things you can do to prepare:

- **Collect Papers:** Find any medical records or reports from past doctors.
- **Make a Timeline:** Write down when the person learned things like walking or talking, and note any delays.
- **Think About Strengths and Weaknesses:** Consider what the person is good at and what might be harder for them.
- **Write Down Questions:** Have any questions you want to ask the team ready.

What to Expect During the Assessment

There might be a few appointments spread out over time. The person might take tests, talk to the team, and be observed. You might also be interviewed.

Getting the Results

Once the tests are done, the team will meet with you to explain what they found. They might give a diagnosis of ID, or they might say the person does not have ID. They will explain why they think this.

What Happens After Diagnosis

A diagnosis is a good thing because it helps get the person the support they need. This support could be things like special education programs, therapy, or job training.

Importance of this Assessment

An ID assessment can be confusing, but it is important. By preparing and talking openly with the team, you can make the process smoother. The diagnosis is the first step to helping the person with ID live a happy and fulfilling life.

COMMON EMOTIONS PARENTS EXPERIENCE

Feeling Upset After an ID Diagnosis? Here is How to Cope

Finding out your child has Intellectual Disability (ID) can be really tough. It is normal to feel shocked, sad, scared, or even angry. Everyone feels differently, and that is okay.

Here are some of those feelings you might have:

- **Shock:** You might not believe it at first. That is okay. Take time to think about it.
- **Sadness:** You might feel like you are missing out on something. It is okay to feel sad.
- **Scared:** You might worry about the future. There is help available, so you do not have to be scared alone.
- **Angry:** You might feel angry at the world or yourself. It is okay to feel angry, but try to find healthy ways to express it.

Here are some things that can help you feel better:

- **Talk to Someone:** Find other parents who have children with ID. They understand how you feel and can offer support.

- **Learn More:** The more you know about ID, the less scary it will seem. Talk to your doctor or therapist and find trusted resources online.
- **Focus on the Good:** Your child has strengths too. Celebrate their achievements and all the things they are good at.
- **Take Care of Yourself:** Eating healthy, getting enough sleep, and doing things you enjoy will help you cope.
- **Get Help:** A therapist can help you manage your feelings and develop coping strategies.

Remember, you are not alone. There are people who can help you and your child. With love, support, and a little time, things will get easier.

FINDING SUPPORT AND BUILDING A COMMUNITY

Finding Support After Your Child's ID Diagnosis

Getting an Intellectual Disability (ID) diagnosis for your child can feel lonely. You might be scared and unsure where to turn for help. But you do not have to go through this alone. There are many people who understand what you are feeling and can offer support.

Why Support Matters

Taking care of a child with ID can be tough. Having a support system lets you share your feelings and worries with people who get it. Support groups are safe places to talk about your emotions, ask questions, and learn from others. They can also help you feel less alone.

Finding Support

There are many ways to find support after an ID diagnosis:

- **Parent Support Groups:** These groups connect parents with children who have ID. You can share experiences, advice, and concerns. There might be national groups with local chapters, or smaller groups run by professionals or experienced parents in your community.

- **Online Communities:** These are online forums and social media groups where parents can connect and share resources from home.
- **Professional Support:** Therapists or counselors can help you manage your emotions and develop ways to communicate with your child. They can also help you and your family deal with the feelings that come with the diagnosis.

Building a Supportive Community

Beyond support, building a community for yourself and your child is important. This helps your child feel like they belong and see positive examples of others with ID. Here are some ways to build a community:

- **Disability Advocacy Organizations:** These connect families, raise awareness about ID, and fight for the rights of people with ID. You can volunteer or participate in events to connect with others.
- **Sibling Support Groups:** Siblings of children with ID can face unique challenges. These groups allow them to connect with others who understand and offer support.
- **Inclusive Activities and Programs:** Look for sports teams, clubs, or activities designed to be

inclusive for people with disabilities. These offer social interaction, skill development, and a sense of belonging.

Standing Up for Your Child

As you raise your child, you will become their advocate. Building a community can help you fight for inclusive education, accessible services, and equal opportunities for your child and others with ID.

Remember, You Are Not Alone

Finding support and building a community are key to coping with an ID diagnosis. By reaching out for help, you will connect with others who understand, build a network of resources, and feel empowered to advocate for your child. You can do this.

2. UNDERSTANDING THE SPECTRUM

Understanding Different Levels of Intellectual Disability (ID)

ID is a condition that affects how someone learns and does daily activities. It starts before age 18 and lasts a lifetime. There are different levels of ID, and each one needs different kinds of help.

IQ Scores and Daily Living Skills

IQ tests measure how well someone learns and solves problems. But ID is also about daily living skills, like dressing, eating, and talking to others. Doctors look at both IQ and daily living skills to figure out the level of ID.

The Four Levels of ID

Here is a simple breakdown of the main levels of ID:

- **Mild ID (IQ: 50-69):** This is most common. People with mild ID learn slower than others, but with help they can:
    - Learn basic reading, writing, and math
    - Talk and understand others
    - Live on their own with some support
    - Have jobs with some supervision

- **Moderate ID (IQ: 35-51):** People with moderate ID need more help in most daily activities. They may:
  - Learn basic communication skills
  - Take care of themselves like dressing and using the bathroom
  - Get job training for specific tasks
  - Need help with where they live and work
- **Severe ID (IQ: 20-35):** People with severe ID need a lot of help with everything. They may:
  - Have little or no talking skills
  - Need help with all daily activities
  - Benefit from programs that teach basic life skills
  - Need constant care from caregivers
- **Profound ID (IQ: Below 20):** This is the rarest type. People with profound ID need constant care and may:
  - Have little to no communication skills
  - Need help with everything all the time
  - Benefit from special therapies

Remember: These are just categories, and people with the same level of ID can have different strengths and challenges. The impact of ID can also depend on the support someone gets, their education, and their unique personality.

Helping People with Different Types of ID

The type of help someone with ID needs depends on the level of their disability. Here are some examples:

- **Mild ID:** Support with school, learning social skills, and job training can help people with mild ID live independently.
- **Moderate and Severe ID:** Special schools, communication therapy, and daily living skills training can help people with moderate and severe ID develop their abilities and have fulfilling lives.
- **Profound ID:** Special therapies that focus on comfort and basic needs are important for people with profound ID.

Looking Beyond Labels

Understanding the levels of ID can help us plan the right kind of support. But it is important to remember that everyone with ID is an individual. Focusing on their strengths, interests, and personality is key to helping them reach their full potential and creating a world where everyone feels included.

Understanding How Intellectual Disability (ID) Affects Development

Every child with ID is different, but there are some general ways it can affect their development. Here is a breakdown of how ID might show up in a child:

Learning: Kids with ID might learn things slower than other kids. They might have trouble reading, writing, and doing math.

Problem-Solving: Figuring things out and making decisions can be harder for kids with ID. They might need more help with things like puzzles or games.

Memory: Remembering things can be tricky for kids with ID. They might forget things they just learned or have trouble remembering instructions.

Talking: Some kids with ID might start talking later than others, or they might have trouble speaking clearly. They might also have trouble understanding what other people are saying.

Social Skills: Making friends and playing with others can be hard for kids with ID. They might not understand the rules of games or how to take turns. They might also have trouble understanding other people's feelings.

Following Directions: Understanding what adults are asking them to do can be a challenge for kids with ID. They might need things explained in a simpler way or need more time to follow instructions.

Physical Development: Some kids with ID might have delays in how their bodies develop. This could mean trouble walking, running, or using their hands well. They might also be more sensitive to sights, sounds, or textures than other kids.

Important to Remember:

- Not every child with ID will have trouble with all these things. Some kids might have more challenges in one area than another.
- The severity of these challenges can vary depending on the type of ID a child has.
- The earlier a child with ID gets help, the better. Doctors and therapists can create a plan to help the child learn and grow in the best way possible.

With the right support, kids with ID can learn, grow, and have fulfilling lives.

EMPOWERING THE CHILD WITH INTELLECTUAL DISABILITY

Every Child with ID has Unique Abilities

Intellectual disability (ID) can affect how a child learns and does daily activities. But even though kids with ID share some things, they are all unique. This article explains why these differences matter.

A World of Unique People

Some things might be similar for kids with ID, but how they experience them can be very different. Here is why:

- **Thinking and Learning:** IQ scores are just one way to measure how someone thinks. Kids with ID might be strong in some areas, like remembering things or being good with puzzles, even if they have trouble with others, like reading or math. Knowing their strengths helps teachers create lessons that work best for them.
- **Talking and Listening:** Some kids with ID might have trouble talking, while others might use special ways to communicate, like sign language or pictures. Knowing how a child communicates best helps us understand them and build a connection.
- **Playing with Others:** Making friends can be hard for kids with ID, but they might all have different reasons. Some might want to play but not know how to ask, while others might prefer to be

alone sometimes. Figuring out what each child likes helps us create ways for them to have fun with others.

- **Learning New Things:** Every child learns in their own way, and this is especially true for kids with ID. Some might learn best by doing things with their hands, while others might need more structure and pictures to help them understand. Knowing a child's learning style helps teachers create lessons that are interesting and effective.

Finding their strength

Focusing only on what is hard can make us forget how amazing kids with ID can be. Finding their strengths is important because it can:

- **Make Them Feel Good:** When we celebrate what a child does well, it shows them they are capable. This helps them feel confident and want to try new things.
- **Help Them Do More on Their Own:** By building on their strengths, kids with ID can learn to do things by themselves. This makes them feel more independent and prouder.
- **Help Them Learn Even More:** A child's strengths can be a starting point to learn new things. For instance, a child who loves music can learn math by using patterns or songs.

Helping Each Child Shine

Knowing how each child is different is key to helping them reach their full potential. Here is how:

- **Special Help Tailored Just for Them:** There is no one-size-fits-all approach. By understanding a child's unique needs, strengths, and learning style, teachers can create special help plans that work best for them.
- **Feeling Welcome Everywhere:** When we celebrate everyone's differences, it makes schools and communities more inclusive. This means everyone feels like they belong and can contribute something special.
- **Reaching for the Stars:** When we help kids with ID build on their strengths, they can achieve amazing things. Special programs that focus on their strengths can help them develop skills, follow their dreams, and live happy, fulfilling lives.

Remember: Every child with ID is special in their own way. By recognizing and celebrating their differences, we can help them succeed and create a world where everyone can thrive.

MythBusters: Busting Common Myths About Intellectual Disability (ID)

Many people misunderstand what Intellectual Disability (ID) is. This article clears up some of the most common myths so we can create a more accepting world for everyone.

Myth 1: People with ID are not smart and cannot learn.

Not true. While ID can make learning slower, everyone with ID has their own strengths and talents. They might be amazing at remembering things, good with puzzles, or really artistic. With the right kind of help and teaching, people with ID can learn and develop new skills their whole lives.

Myth 2: ID is a mental illness.

This is not right. ID is a different kind of developmental condition. People with ID can have mental health problems just like anyone else, but these are separate things that need different treatments.

Myth 3: People with ID are violent.

Not true at all. Studies show no connection between ID and violence. In fact, people with ID are more likely to be the victims of crime than the criminals themselves. Sometimes they might act out because they are frustrated or cannot communicate well, but there are ways to help them manage those feelings.

Myth 4: People with ID cannot live on their own.

It depends. The amount of help someone with ID needs depends on how severe their disability is. With the right support and training, many people with ID can live independently or with some help, and even contribute to their communities.

Myth 5: Kids with ID will outgrow it.

Not exactly. ID is a lifelong condition. But with early intervention and ongoing support, people with ID can learn a lot and reach their full potential. Early help can make a big difference in their lives and future opportunities.

Why These Myths Matter

Believing these myths can hurt people with ID in a few ways:

- **Missed chances:** If people think someone with ID cannot learn, they might not get the education or jobs they deserve.

- **Feeling left out:** Negative stereotypes can make people with ID feel isolated and unwelcome.
- **Lack of Support:** If people do not understand the needs of people with ID, there might not be enough programs or services to help them succeed.

Building a Better World of Inclusivity

By learning the facts about ID, we can create a more inclusive and supportive world for everyone:

- **Focus on what they can do:** Highlighting the strengths and abilities of people with ID helps them feel good about themselves and what they can achieve.
- **Spread the word:** Educating others about ID can challenge stereotypes and create a more understanding environment.
- **Celebrate Differences:** Everyone has something special to offer, and people with ID are no exception. Their unique strengths make our communities richer.

Remember: ID is a complex condition, but by understanding it better, we can create a world where everyone has the chance to succeed and live a happy life. Let us celebrate the full range of human experiences and the potential within each person.

3. BEYOND THE LABEL

Finding the Strengths and interests

Many times, we focus on what can be hard for people with Intellectual Disability (ID). But what about the amazing things they can do? This article explains why focusing on strengths is important.

Looking Beyond Challenges

Everyone with ID has challenges, but they also have strengths and talents that we might miss. These strengths can be in many areas:

- **Creativity:** People with ID might be great at art, music, or dance. Their unique way of seeing the world can lead to amazing and creative things.
- **Solving Problems:** Sometimes, people with ID can find different ways to do things, or solve problems in unexpected ways.
- **Being Social:** People with ID can be very caring and understanding. They might be really good at making friends or helping others feel good.
- **Physical Skills:** Some people with ID are strong, coordinated, or have a great sense of rhythm. These talents can help them with sports or other activities.

Discover What They Love

Everyone feels good when they can do something they enjoy. This is especially true for people with ID. Here is why finding their interests is important:

- **Wanting to Do More:** When people with ID can do things they like, they are more motivated and want to keep doing them. This helps them feel proud of themselves.
- **Learning New Things:** Doing things they love can help people with ID learn new skills or get better at things they already know.
- **Feeling Happy:** Doing fun activities helps people with ID feel good about themselves. It gives them a way to express themselves and relax.

Helping Them Shine

There are ways to help people with ID discover their strengths and interests:

- **Watching Closely:** Pay attention to what they seem to enjoy doing, what they are good at, or what activities they keep coming back to.
- **Trying New Things:** Give them opportunities to try new activities, join different clubs, or explore different hobbies.

- **Special Tests:** Sometimes, there are tests that can help identify a person's strengths, how they learn best, and what areas they might be talented in.
- **Talking it Out:** Talk to the person with ID, their caregivers, and teachers. They might have great ideas about the person's interests and goals.

Building on Strengths

Once we know what someone with ID is good at and what they enjoy, we can help them reach their full potential:

- **Special Programs:** Create learning programs that focus on their strengths and interests. This will make learning more fun and engaging.
- **Job Training:** Help them develop skills related to their interests so they can get jobs they will enjoy and feel successful in.
- **Activities with Friends:** Find activities related to their interests that they can do with others. This helps them feel included and make friends.

The Power of Strengths

Focusing on strengths is a big change in how we think about ID. By finding what people with ID are good at and what they love, we can help them:

- Discover their potential: They can see how much they can achieve.
- Find joy in what they do: They can have fun and feel good about themselves.
- Be a part of their community: They can contribute their skills and talents and feel like they belong.

Let us celebrate the abilities of everyone, including people with ID. There is potential in everyone, and focusing on strengths paves the way for a happier and more fulfilling life for all.

Creating self-esteem and confidence

People with Intellectual Disability (ID) can sometimes feel down on themselves. This article talks about ways to help them feel good about who they are.

Why Confidence Matters

There are a few reasons why feeling good about themselves is important for people with ID:

- **Focus on what they can do:** When we focus on what is hard for them, it can make them feel like they cannot do anything. But everyone is good at something. Helping them find their strengths makes them feel proud.

- **Trying new things:** Feeling confident makes people want to try new things and learn new skills. This can help them do more and be more independent.
- **Making friends:** When people feel good about themselves, it is easier to make friends and feel like they belong.

Helping Them Shine

Here are some things we can do to help people with ID build confidence:

- **Celebrate their wins.** No matter how small, acknowledging their achievements shows them they are doing a good job and keeps them motivated.
- **Let them do things for themselves:** Helping them learn to do things like dressing themselves or making their own lunch builds confidence in their abilities.
- **Positive words:** Tell them they are doing a good job and focus on the effort they put in, not just the outcome.
- **Let them choose:** Giving them choices, even small ones, shows you trust them and helps them feel in control.

The Power of Friends and Family

The people around someone with ID can really make a difference in their confidence:

- **Supportive family and friends:** Having people who care about them and believe in them is important for everyone.
- **Role models:** Meeting successful people with ID can show them what is possible and inspire them to reach their goals.
- **Speaking up for themselves:** Teaching them to ask for what they need and express themselves helps them feel confident and in control of their lives.

Making a Plan of Action

Here are some ways to put these ideas into action:

- **Special plans:** Create a plan with specific goals for each person, based on their strengths and what they want to achieve.
- **Learning new skills:** Help them learn skills that will be helpful in everyday life, like communication or problem-solving.
- **Positive talk:** Always use kind and encouraging words when talking to them.

- **Making choices:** Give them opportunities to make small choices throughout the day so they feel like they have some control.

Building confidence takes time, but it is worth it

By focusing on their strengths, celebrating their achievements, and helping them build positive relationships, we can empower people with ID to feel good about themselves and reach their full potential. Everyone deserves to feel confident and capable, no matter their abilities.

Embracing your child's individuality

Being a parent of a child with Intellectual Disability (ID) is special. It is about finding the beauty in their unique way of seeing the world. While ID can be tough, it also makes your child who they are, and that is something to celebrate.

Every Child is Different

ID is not the same for everyone. Just like other kids, children with ID have their own personalities, interests, and little quirks. It is important to see your child as a whole person, not just a diagnosis.

Celebrating Their Specialness

Here are ways to celebrate your child's unique personality:

- **Loving What They Love:** Does your child love dinosaurs or making music? Let them explore their passions, no matter what they are. This makes them feel happy and proud.
- **Their Special Things:** Maybe your child loves a certain color or has a funny way of saying things. That is okay. These quirks make them special.
- **What They are Good At:** Every child is good at something, even if it is different from other kids. Find what your child is good at and help them get even better.
- **Listening to Them:** Let your child express themselves, however they can. This helps you understand them better and see their unique personality.

Helping Them Feel Good About Themselves

By celebrating your child's personality, you help them feel good about who they are. Here is how:

- **Positive Words:** Tell your child you are proud of them, no matter how big or small their accomplishment. This makes them want to keep trying new things.

- **Celebrating Every Step:** Focus on how much your child has learned, not where they need to be. This shows them they are doing a great job.
- **Breaking Stereotypes:** Do not let others bring your child down. Being different is a strength, not a weakness.

Building a Happy Place for Them to Grow

Your child will grow best in a loving and supportive environment:

- **Activities for Everyone:** Find activities where all kinds of kids can join in. This helps your child make friends and feel included.
- **Role Models:** Show your child people with ID who are successful. This shows them they can achieve their dreams too.
- **Talking it Out:** Make your home a safe space where your child feels comfortable being themselves.

The Most Beautiful Song

Raising a child with ID is a special journey. By celebrating their unique personality, helping them feel good about themselves, and creating a supportive environment, you are helping them reach their full potential. Remember, the most beautiful music comes from instruments that all sound a little different. Embrace the special song of your child's individuality.

Setting goals and achieving dreams

Some people with ID face challenges, but that does not mean they cannot have a great life. Setting goals can help them get where they want to be.

Why Setting Goals Matters

Goals are like a roadmap. They help people with ID know what they are working towards and give them a reason to keep trying. Here is why setting goals is important:

- **Feeling Motivated:** Goals make people with ID want to work hard because they know what they are trying to achieve.
- **Feeling Confident:** When people with ID reach their goals, it makes them feel good about themselves and believe they can do anything.
- **Doing Things Themselves:** Goals can be about learning new skills to do things by themselves, like cooking or cleaning. This makes them feel more independent.

- **Happy and Healthy Life:** Goals can be about things that make people happy and healthy, like making friends or joining a sports team.

Setting Goals that You Can Reach

The best goals for people with ID are ones they can actually achieve. Here are some tips:

- **Pick things they are good at:** If someone is good at drawing, maybe their goal can be to win a local art contest.
- **Start small and grow:** Big goals can be overwhelming. Break them down into smaller steps so they do not seem so scary.
- **Goals for Everyone:** Goals should be based on what the person with ID wants, not what others think they should do.
- **Work Together:** Parents, teachers, and therapists can help people with ID set goals that are just right.

Following Your Dreams

Everyone has dreams, and people with ID are no different. Having a dream can be a powerful thing:

- **Inspiration to Try:** Dreams can make people with ID want to try new things and reach for something bigger.

- **Believing in Yourself:** Working towards a dream shows people with ID that they can achieve great things.
- **Feeling Good About Life:** Having a dream gives people with ID a reason to feel hopeful and excited about the future.

Helping Dreams Come True

Here are some ways to help people with ID chase their dreams:

- **Talk about Dreams:** Listen to what people with ID want to achieve and help them figure out how to get there.
- **Help Overcome Challenges:** There might be things that make it hard to reach a dream. Help find ways to overcome those challenges.
- **Celebrate Every Step:** Even small steps towards a dream are important. Celebrate their progress to keep them motivated.
- **Be Their Champion:** Help people with ID find the resources and support they need to make their dreams a reality.

Conclusion

Living a happy life with ID is not about being perfect. It is about finding what you are good at, setting goals you can reach, and following your dreams. With a little help and support, everyone can achieve their goals and live a life filled with meaning and purpose. Every journey starts with a first step, and anything is possible with hard work and a dream.

4. NAVIGATING THE EDUCATIONAL SYSTEM

Finding the Best School

Every child with ID learns differently. This article will help you pick the right school for your child's special needs. There are 3 main choices: public schools, private schools, and special programs.

Public Schools

- **Good for:** Making friends with other kids, getting extra help (IEPs), learning life skills (like speech therapy).
- **Things to Consider:** Large classes can make it hard for teachers to focus on each child. There may not be enough teachers specially trained to help kids with ID.

Private Schools

- **Good for:** Smaller classes with more attention, specialized programs for ID, experienced teachers.
- **Things to Consider:** Private schools can be expensive, and there may not be one near you. Your child might not get as much chance to make friends with kids who do not have ID.

Special Programs

- **Good for:** Children who need a lot of extra help, learning practical skills for daily life, getting therapy like occupational therapy.
- **Things to Consider:** There may be a waiting list to get into these programs. They might focus more on life skills than regular school subjects. Your child might not have many opportunities to interact with other kids.

The Best Choice for Your Child

The best school depends on your child's needs. Here are some things to think about:

- How much help does your child need?
- How does your child learn best?
- Does your child like to be around other kids?
- What are your goals for your child's future?

The Most Important Thing

The most important thing is to find a school where your child feels good and can learn. Talk to the teachers and see if it feels like a good fit for your child.

Individualized Education Plans (IEPs)

Your child just got diagnosed with ID. It can be a lot to handle, but there is help available at school. An IEP is a special plan to help your child succeed.

What is an IEP?

An IEP is like a map for your child's education. It shows what your child needs to learn and how they will learn it best. Here is how it works:

- **The School Checks Your Child:** First, the school will test your child to see what kind of help they need.
- **The IEP Meeting:** Then, you will meet with the teachers and other helpers to create a plan. This plan will include:

    o   What your child is good at
    o   What your child needs to work on
    o   Extra help your child might need in school (like speech therapy)

- **Making Changes:** The plan can change throughout the year as your child learns new things. You will meet again to talk about how your child is doing.

How to Get the Most Out of Their IEP

- **Learn About Your Rights:** There is a law called IDEA that says all kids with disabilities deserve a good education. Learn about it so you know what to ask for.
- **Gather Information:** Think about what helps your child learn best. Are they good at drawing? Do they learn best by listening or doing? This will help make the IEP stronger.
- **Be Involved:** The IEP meeting is your chance to speak up for your child. Ask questions and tell the teachers what you think is important.
- **Focus on What Your Child Can Do:** Tell the teachers about your child's strengths. The IEP should help them learn even more.
- **Set Goals:** The IEP should have goals that your child can reach. These goals will help them track their progress and feel proud of themselves.
- **Stay Informed:** Talk to your child's teachers regularly. Ask them how the IEP is working and if anything needs to change.

You Are Your Child's Best Helper.

The IEP can make a big difference in your child's education. By being involved and working with the teachers, you can help your child reach their full potential.

Early Intervention Programs

When a child has ID, it can be scary. But there is good news. Special programs can help them learn and grow right from the start. These programs are called "early intervention."

Why Early Intervention Matters

A young child's brain is like a sponge, soaking up new things all the time. Early intervention programs take advantage of this by giving your child extra help during this important time. Here is how it can benefit your child:

- **Learning More:** These programs can help your child learn new things like talking, remembering, and solving problems. They make learning fun with games and activities.
- **Talking and Playing with Others:** These programs help your child interact with other kids. This teaches them social skills and how to manage their emotions.
- **Taking Care of Themselves:** These programs can help your child learn to do things for themselves, like dressing and eating. This makes them feel more independent.
- **Fewer Frustrations:** These programs can help your child understand the world around them

better. This can lead to fewer meltdowns and bad behavior.

Benefits for the Whole Family

Early intervention is not just good for your child. It helps parents too.

- **Learning How to Help:** These programs teach parents how to support their child's development at home.
- **Feeling Less Stressed:** Seeing your child progress can make you feel less worried and overwhelmed.
- **Finding Support:** These programs connect families with other parents and resources that can help.

Investing in a Brighter Future

Early intervention is like planting a seed. The sooner you plant it, the bigger and stronger the plant will grow. Here is why it is important:

- **Happier and Healthier Life:** Early intervention can help your child live a happier, healthier life by giving them the skills they need to be independent.

- **Saving Money:** These programs can save money in the long run by reducing the need for extra help later on.
- **A More Inclusive World:** When everyone has the opportunity to learn and grow, our communities become stronger and more welcoming.

Getting Your Child Started

If your child has ID, talk to your doctor about early intervention programs. They can help you find the right program for your child.

Remember, early intervention can make a big difference in your child's life. By getting them the help they need early on, you can help them reach their full potential and shine bright.

Getting Help Early

The first few years of life are very important for learning and growing. This is especially true for children with ID. Getting help early can make a big difference.

Why Early Intervention Matters

- A young child's brain is like a sponge, learning new things quickly. Early intervention programs take advantage of this to give your child extra help during this important time.
- These programs can help your child learn new skills like talking, playing with others, and taking care of themselves. This can lead to fewer tantrums and a happier child.

How to Get Help

- Talk to your child's doctor if you have any concerns about their development. The doctor can refer you to a program that can help.
- There will be a meeting to see if your child qualifies for the program.
- If they do qualify, a plan will be made to help your child reach their goals.

What You Can Do to Help

- Go to all the meetings and therapy sessions with your child.
- Ask questions if you do not understand something.
- Practice the things your child learns in therapy at home.
- There are also parent support groups that can help you connect with other families facing similar challenges.

Early Help Means a Brighter Future

By getting your child with ID into an early intervention program early, you can help them reach their full potential and live a happy and fulfilling life.

Transition services: Preparing for the future beyond high school

High school graduation is a big deal. But for young adults with ID, it can be a little scary. There are new things to learn like living on their own, getting a job, and being part of the community. Transition services can help.

What are Transition Services?

It is a fancy way of saying "getting ready for life after high school." These programs help young adults with ID learn important skills like:

- **Taking care of themselves:** This includes things like cooking, cleaning, and doing laundry.
- **Getting a job:** They can help with finding a job, writing a resume, and preparing for interviews.
- **Living on their own:** This could mean learning how to use public transportation, manage money, and be a good roommate.

- **Making friends:** Transition services can help young adults find social activities and connect with others.

Why is it Important?

Transition services help young adults with ID become more independent and confident. This means they can live on their own, get a job, and do the things they want to do.

How to Get Help

Talk to your child's teacher or counselor before they graduate high school. They can help you find transition services in your area.

What You Can Do to Help

- Go to meetings with your child about transition services.
- Help your child practice the skills they are learning.
- Encourage your child to be involved in making decisions about their future.

A Bright Future

Transition services can help your child with ID have a happy and fulfilling life after high school.

5. BUILDING YOUR TEAM

Doctors: Pediatricians, neurologists, and specialists for specific needs.

- Main Doctor: Pediatrician
    - Does checkups, gives shots, monitors growth.
    - Treats common illnesses.
    - Manages other health problems or refers to specialists.
- Brain Doctor: Neurologist
    - Helps find the cause of ID (in some cases).
    - Manages seizures, tremors, or movement problems.
    - Does tests on thinking and movement.
- Other Specialists (depending on needs):
    - Developmental pediatrician: helps with learning and growing.
    - Speech therapist: helps with communication.
    - Occupational therapist: helps with daily activities (dressing, eating).
    - Physical therapist: helps with movement.
    - Behavioral specialist: helps manage challenging behaviors.
- Working Together for Best Care:
    - Talk openly with all doctors and share questions or concerns.

- o Make sure all doctors have your child's medical records.
- o Have meetings with doctors together to discuss progress as a team.
- Remember: You are your child's best helper.
  - o The more you know, the better you can advocate for their health.
  - o Working together as a team ensures your child gets the care they need.

Therapists: Occupational therapists, speech-language pathologists, and physical therapists.

- Occupational Therapist (OT) helps with daily activities:
  - o Dressing, eating, playing.
  - o Getting used to different sensations (touch, sound, light).
  - o Recommending tools or technology for more independence.
- Speech-Language Pathologist (SLP) helps with communication:
  - o Speaking and understanding language.
  - o Using pictures, devices, or social skills to communicate.
  - o Making friends through conversation.
- Physical Therapist (PT) helps with movement:
  - o Getting stronger and improving coordination.

- o Learning to walk, run, and play.
  - o Recommending equipment for safe movement.
- Therapists work together as a team:
  - o Discuss child's progress and plan care.
  - o Teach you exercises and strategies to help at home.

Remember: You are your child's biggest champion. By working together with therapists, you can help your child with ID thrive.

Social workers: Connecting families to resources and support services

- Social workers help families with children with ID by:
  - o Talking about your child's needs and your family's needs (money, emotions, support).
  - o Connecting you with resources (financial help, childcare, programs, therapy).
  - o Helping you fight for your child's rights (at school, doctor's appointments, government).
  - o Connecting you with other families who understand.
  - o Helping you during tough times (when your child gets older or has challenging behaviors).

- Social workers do more than connect you:
    - o Teach you how to help your child grow and be more independent (communication, managing behavior).
    - o Help you talk to your child's teachers, therapists, and doctors (ensure everyone works together).
    - o Help you plan for your child's future (living arrangements, jobs, money management).
- Working together is best:
    - o Talk openly and honestly about your concerns and questions.
    - o Work together to set goals for your child and family.
    - o Respect each other (you are a team working for the same goal: helping your child thrive).

Remember: Social workers are there to support you and your child on your journey with ID. They can help you find resources, advocate for your rights, and build a brighter future for your child. You are not alone.

Working Together as a Team

Why it is important:

- Doctors & therapists learn more by sharing information (better care plan).
- Everyone focuses on their strengths (avoids extra work).
- Less confusion and better trust with clear communication.
- Problems get spotted earlier with regular talks.
- Best ideas from everyone create the most helpful plan.

How to make it easier:

- Regular meetings to discuss progress.
- Easy ways for everyone to contact and share information.
- Keep all information in one place for easy access.
- Treat each other with respect and value everyone's contribution.
- Include the person with ID and family in discussions and decisions.
- Discuss disagreements calmly and respectfully.

Technology can help:

- Websites and apps for information sharing and scheduling meetings.
- Video calls for appointments can improve attendance.

The result:

- Working together creates the best care plan for a happy and fulfilling life.
- Everyone has something important to offer, and together you create the best outcome.

6. THE POWER OF ADVOCACY

Understanding your child's rights and entitlements

When your child has ID, you might worry about their future. But there is good news. They have rights that give them access to things they need to learn and grow.

The Law Says Your Child Can Get a Free Education

- A law called IDEA says all children with disabilities, including ID, must get a free public education in a regular classroom whenever possible.
- This education should be planned just for your child's needs.
- Your child has the right to be tested to see if they qualify for this special help.

There are Other Laws to Help Your Child Too

- Another law, the ADA, says no one can discriminate against your child because of their ID. This means they can use public places, transportation, and even talk on the phone.

- There are programs that can help your child find a job, get health insurance, and even find an affordable place to live.
- Some programs can even give your family money to help with your child's care.

How to Find Out What Your Child Qualifies For

- Talk to your child's doctor, teachers, and social worker. They can help you understand your child's needs and what programs they might qualify for.
- There are also organizations that advocate for disability rights. They can give you information and help you fight for your child's rights.

You Are Your Child's Biggest Champion.

The more you know about your child's rights, the better you can advocate for them. Here are some tips:

- Learn about the laws that can help your child.
- Gather documents that show your child's needs.
- Ask questions and do not be afraid to speak up.
- Go to meetings about your child's education and care.
- Get to know the people who work with your child.

Working Together for a Brighter Future

By understanding your child's rights, you can help them get the support they need to live a happy and fulfilling life. Remember, you are not alone. There are laws and programs in place to help your child reach their full potential.

Effective communication with educators and healthcare providers

Helping Your Child (ID) Speak Up for Themselves

When your child has ID, it can be hard for them to tell you what they want or need. But there are ways to help them learn to speak up for themselves. This is called self-advocacy.

Building Confidence to Speak Up

- Help your child feel good about themselves. Let them know you are proud of them and their efforts.
- Talk openly and honestly with your child. Let them tell you how they feel and what they think.
- Give your child choices throughout the day. This could be things like what to wear or what to eat for

a snack. As they get better at making choices, give them harder ones.

- Be a good example. Show your child how to speak up for yourself by telling people what you need.

Helping Your Child Practice Speaking Up

- Start with small things. Maybe your child can ask for a drink when they are thirsty.
- Act out different situations with your child. Practice how they can ask for something they need or tell someone how they feel.
- Make stories together that show how to talk to people in different situations.
- Use pictures or symbols to help your child communicate if talking is hard.
- Praise your child every time they try to speak up for themselves, even if they do not get what they want.
- Help your child use "I" statements. This means saying things like "I feel tired" instead of "This is boring."

Growing Independence

As your child gets better at speaking up, encourage them to do more things on their own:

- Teach your child how to ask for help when they need it.
- Help your child tell people their preferences in school, therapy, or other places.
- Give your child choices whenever you can. This could be about what to wear, what to do after school, or what game to play.

Remember

- It is important for your child to be polite while speaking up for themselves.
- Not everyone will always say yes to what your child wants. Help them learn how to deal with disappointment.

By helping your child practice self-advocacy, you are giving them the tools they need to live a happy and independent life.

Building partnerships with schools and community organizations

When your child has ID, you might worry about school and how they will fit in with others. But there are many people who can help. Here is how to work with schools and community groups to give your child the best support possible.

Why Working Together is Important

- Schools and community groups have different ways to help your child. By working together, they can offer more complete support.
- This support can go beyond just schoolwork. It can help your child make friends, learn new skills, and feel like they belong.
- Schools and community groups can also help your child prepare for adulthood, like learning job skills or how to live independently.
- The more you talk to the people who work with your child, the more they can understand your child's needs.

Finding People to Help

- At School: Look for teachers who work with students with ID, counselors, and social workers.

There might also be a parent-teacher association (PTA) you can connect with.

- In the Community: There are groups that advocate for disability rights, offer fun activities after school, teach job skills, or can help your child live on their own someday. You might also find support groups at your house of worship.

How to Build Strong Relationships

- Talk to the people who work with your child and tell them about your child's strengths, challenges, and goals.
- Be open and honest about your concerns.
- Treat everyone with respect and remember that you are all working towards the same goal: helping your child succeed.
- Have regular meetings to discuss your child's progress and make plans together.
- You can also organize events to bring families, teachers, and community members together to learn from each other.

Using Technology to Stay Connected

- There are websites and apps that can help schools, families, and community groups share information and stay organized.

- These tools can also be used to store information about your child's progress and goals so everyone has easy access.

Remember

By working together with schools and community groups, you can create a strong support system for your child. This network of people can help your child learn, grow, and reach their full potential.

7. UNLOCKING POTENTIAL

Learning styles

- Every child learns differently, including children with ID.
- There are 4 main learning styles:
    - Seeing things (pictures, charts, videos)
    - Hearing things (instructions, stories)
    - Doing things (moving around, activities)
    - Learning with others (working together)
- How to find out your child's learning style:
    - Watch what they enjoy (looking at books, listening to music, playing games)
    - Talk to their teachers and therapists
    - Try different activities
- Tips for helping your child learn:
    - Seeing: use pictures, charts, and videos
    - Hearing: read aloud, audiobooks, podcasts, songs, rhymes
    - Doing: games, puzzles, hands-on activities
    - Learning with others: group work, partner work
- Other tips:
    - Find things they like to learn about
    - Praise their effort
    - Give them a routine
    - Break down big tasks into smaller steps

- Be patient and try different things to find the best way for your child to learn.

Effective teaching strategies

- Here are 3 ways to help people with ID learn:

  o Pictures and Charts:
    - Use pictures instead of words to explain things.
    - Start with simple pictures and make them more complex later.
    - Use different types of pictures like matching games.
  o Learning by Doing:
    - Teach through activities instead of just talking.
    - This helps them learn with their bodies, not just listen.
    - Break down skills into small steps and show them how to do it first.
  o Repetition:
    - People with ID may need more practice than others.
    - The more they practice, the better they learn.
    - Make practice fun and celebrate their improvements.

Remember:

- Everyone learns differently, find what works best for them.
- Be patient and positive, learning takes time.
- Celebrate even small improvements to keep them motivated.

Differentiated instruction

- Every child with ID learns differently, regular teaching methods might not be the best.
- Here is how teachers and caregivers can help:
    - Find their learning style: See if they learn best by seeing pictures, doing activities, or listening.
    - Make learning different for each child: Use shorter assignments, different ways to answer questions, etc.
    - Change how they show what they know: Let them draw pictures, build with blocks, etc. instead of writing long answers.
    - Work in small groups: Help them learn from and with other children.
    - Give clear instructions and routines: Help them feel comfortable knowing what to expect.
    - Celebrate small improvements: Motivate them by celebrating their effort.

- o Work with parents and therapists: Learn what works best for them at home and in therapy.
- There is no one-size-fits-all approach. Find what works best for each child to help them succeed.

Celebrating progress and growth

- Celebrate people with ID's achievements, big or small. Here is why:
  - o It makes them feel good and want to keep learning.
  - o It shows them they can do things and builds their confidence.
  - o It makes them feel loved and supported.

What to celebrate:

- School achievements (new skills, projects, good grades)
- Social achievements (making friends, sharing, solving problems)
- Self-care achievements (brushing teeth, dressing, using the bathroom)
- Trying new things (overcoming fears)

How to make celebrations meaningful

- Do something, they enjoy (favorite activity, small gift, hug).
- Praise their effort, not just the result.
- Celebrate with others (family, friends, teachers).
- Make it a tradition (special ways to celebrate).
- Celebrate every step of the way, not just big achievements.

Help people with ID keep growing

- Set goals together to give them direction and control.
- Focus on their strengths to build confidence and motivation.
- Use positive words (talk about progress, use "yet" instead of "cannot").
- Learn from mistakes (use them as a chance to try again).
- Celebrating milestones is about acknowledging their journey and growth. It empowers them to reach their full potential.

8. COMMUNICATION IS KEY

Exploring different communication methods

- Not everyone with ID can talk like most people, but they can still communicate.
- Here are different ways to communicate:
    o Talking (words and sentences)
    o Body language (facial expressions, gestures, eye contact)
    o Pictures and symbols (pointing to what they want)
    o Assistive technology (tablets with pictures, talking devices)
- Find the best way for someone to communicate by considering:
    o Age (younger - pictures, older - more talking)
    o Skills (good at pointing? using facial expressions?)
    o What they prefer (if they can tell you)
- Tips to help people with ID communicate better:
    o Use short and simple words, speak slowly and clearly.
    o Use pictures and gestures to help them understand.
    o Be patient and give them time to respond.
    o Celebrate their efforts.
- Special tools to help people with ID talk:

- o Picture boards (pictures of what they want)
  - o Communication devices (say words or phrases for them)
  - o Computers (type or use pictures to communicate)
- Everyone communicates differently, be patient and understanding. This helps them feel connected to others.

Augmentative and alternative communication (AAC)

- AAC (Augmentative and Alternative Communication) helps people with ID communicate in different ways.
- AAC is important because it lets people with ID:
  - o Feel in control (tell you what they want/need).
  - o Make friends (communicate and connect with others).
  - o Learn new things (by talking and asking questions).
  - o Feel good about themselves (express themselves and feel confident).
- Choosing the right AAC method depends on the person's:
  - o Age (younger - pictures, older - talking devices).
  - o Skills (good at pointing? using gestures?).

- Types of AAC:
    - No tools (facial expressions, gestures, sounds).
    - Low-tech AAC (picture boards, symbol books).
    - High-tech AAC (talking devices).
- Tips to help people with ID use AAC:
    - Start simple (few pictures/symbols at first).
    - Show them how (use the system yourself and let them copy).
    - Be patient (give them time to communicate).
    - Celebrate their efforts.
- Fun AAC tools:
    - Talking devices (say words or phrases).
    - Touchscreens (easy to use).
    - Apps (help learn and practice communication skills).
- Everyone communicates differently, use AAC to help them find a way that works for them. This helps them feel connected to others.

Social communication skills

- Social skills help people with ID get along with others. Here are some social skills:
    - Talking and listening (using words, gestures, facial expressions)

- o Taking turns (knowing when to talk and listen)
  - o Understanding feelings (knowing how someone feels)
  - o Solving problems together (disagreeing in a nice way)
- **How to help people with ID learn social skills:**
  - o Show them how (do it yourself and let them copy).
  - o Practice (act out conversations or pretend).
  - o Join a social skills group (meet and practice with others).
  - o Use pictures and stories (explain social situations).
  - o Celebrate success (praise them for trying).
- **Fun tools to help with social skills:**
  - o Computers and games (special games to learn social skills).
  - o Video chat (talk to friends and family far away).
- **How to make friends:**
  - o Start a conversation (say hi and ask their name).
  - o Take turns talking (do not interrupt).
  - o Be a good listener (pay attention to your friend).
  - o Be kind and helpful (share and offer help).

o Learning social skills helps people with ID make friends and have fun. Everyone deserves to feel like they belong.

Empowering your child to express their wants and needs

- Talking is important for kids with ID because it helps them:
  - o Have fewer meltdowns (express their needs).
  - o Be more independent (ask for things).
  - o Make more friends (communicate with others).
  - o Learn more (talk about new things).
- Some reasons why talking might be hard for kids with ID:
  - o Saying difficult words.
  - o Understanding what others say.
  - o Showing feelings with face and body.
- How to help your child talk more:
  - o Listen closely (even to non-verbal cues).
  - o Use short and simple words, speak slowly and clearly.
  - o Use pictures and gestures to help them communicate and understand.
  - o Celebrate all their efforts to talk.
- Special tools to help talk:

- o Picture boards (pictures of things they want/need).
  - o Sign language (learn some basic signs).
  - o Talking devices (say words or phrases for them).
- Other ways to help:
  - o Make routines (less stress, easier to talk about needs).
  - o Give choices with pictures or objects (feel in control, communicate preferences).
  - o Take turns talking (learn conversation flow).
- Work with others:
  - o Talk to your doctor (find a speech therapist).
  - o Talk to your child's teachers (use same communication strategies at home and school).
  - o Talk to everyone who cares for your child (everyone communicates the same way).
  - o Be patient and understanding, everyone learns at their own pace. By helping your child talk more, they will feel happier and more connected.

Selecting the right AAC system

- AAC systems (picture boards, talking devices) help children with ID communicate when they cannot talk the usual way.
- Choose the talking tool based on your child's:
  - Age (Younger - simple tools, Older - complex tools).
  - Abilities (Can they point? Use a touchscreen?).
  - Learning style (Visual, auditory, kinesthetic).
  - Preferences (Use pictures they like, e.g., animals).
- Types of talking tools:
  - No tools (facial expressions, gestures, sounds).
  - Simple picture boards (pictures of what they want/need).
  - Talking devices (say words or phrases, some with touchscreens).
- Get help choosing:
  - Talk to your doctor (get a speech therapist recommendation).
  - Work with teachers (everyone uses the same tool).
- Be patient. It takes time to learn how to use AAC systems.

- With the right tool, your child can communicate and feel more connected.

Using AAC effectively

- AAC systems (pictures, symbols, talking devices) help kids with ID communicate.
- For AAC to work best, kids need to use it all the time at home and school because:
  - They learn more by practicing with AAC.
  - They can make more friends by communicating with others.
  - They can be more independent by telling you what they want/need.
  - They avoid frustration by being able to communicate.
- How to help your child use AAC at home:
  - Show them how to use it (use it yourself and let them copy).
  - Practice during daily activities (meals, playtime, bedtime).
  - Use pictures and symbols they like.
  - Celebrate their efforts to talk.
- How to help your child use AAC at school:
  - Work with teachers to use AAC the same way as at home.
  - Train teachers on how to use AAC and help your child use it in class.

- o Make AAC system accessible at school (all day, lessons, activities).
- o Have other kids who know AAC show your child how to use it.
- Working together at home and school:
  - o Use picture schedules to show what is coming next (helps them know when to use AAC).
  - o Keep a communication notebook to share information and tips about your child's AAC use.
  - o Talk to teachers often about your child's AAC use and progress.
- When things get tough:
  - o If your child gets frustrated, find out why and make AAC easier to use.
  - o Know how to fix or get help if the AAC system malfunctions.
  - o Keep it fun with games, activities, and apps that work with AAC.
- The more we help at home and school, the better kids with ID can use AAC to talk, feel confident, make friends, and learn. Be patient and celebrate their progress.

Supporting speech development

- AAC and speech therapy can help people with ID learn to speak better.

- Why speaking can be hard for people with ID:
    - Moving their mouth muscles.
    - Understanding language.
    - Learning sounds, words, and grammar.
- How AAC helps people with ID learn to speak:
    - Shows how talking works (word order, sounds).
    - Gives confidence to talk more.
    - Less frustration by expressing themselves.
- How speech therapy helps people with ID learn to speak:
    - Mouth exercises to improve speaking muscles.
    - Learning how to make sounds for words.
    - Building sentences (putting words in order).
- Using AAC and speech therapy together is even better:
    - Therapists can use AAC to practice speech therapy skills.
    - AAC supports speaking even if it is difficult.
    - AAC helps learn the building blocks of speaking.
- Tips:
    - Work together (therapists, teachers, caregivers).
    - Practice talking and using AAC regularly.
    - Celebrate every effort to speak.

- Computers can help too:
    - o Talking devices (help learn how words sound).
    - o Games and apps (help learn to speak and use AAC).
- By using AAC and speech therapy together, people with ID can improve their speaking skills, feel more confident, and connect better with others. Be patient and celebrate their progress.

Encouraging self-advocacy through communication

- Speaking up is important for kids with ID because it helps them:
    - o Do things on their own (by telling you what they need).
    - o Make choices (about things that affect them).
    - o Make more friends (by talking about their feelings).
    - o Have fewer meltdowns (by expressing what bothers them).
- Some reasons why speaking up can be hard for kids with ID:
    - o Saying difficult words.
    - o Understanding others.
    - o Showing feelings with face and body.
- How to help your child speak up for themselves:

- o Listen closely (even to non-verbal cues).
- o Celebrate all their efforts to talk.
- o Use short and simple words, speak slowly and clearly.
- o Use pictures and gestures to help them communicate and understand.
- Special tools to help speak up:
  - o Picture boards (pictures of things they want/need).
  - o Sign language (learn some basic signs).
  - o Talking devices (say words or phrases for them).
- Practice speaking up:
  - o Act out situations and practice how to speak up.
  - o Join social skills groups (learn to talk to others and express themselves).
  - o Use pictures and stories (show how to speak up in different situations).
- Work with others:
  - o Talk to teachers (use same strategies at home and school).
  - o Talk to therapists (improve communication skills and feel comfortable speaking up).
- Be patient and understanding, everyone learns at their own pace. By helping your child speak up, they will feel more confident and in control.

9. BUILDING LIFE SKILLS

Daily routines: Developing self-care skills

- Daily tasks like dressing, bathing, and brushing teeth are important because they help people with ID:
    - Be more independent (do things by themselves).
    - Take care of themselves (stay healthy).
    - Live on their own (in the future).
- Learning daily tasks can be hard for people with ID because:
    - It takes them longer to learn new things.
    - Remembering many steps can be difficult.
    - Some sensations during tasks might feel uncomfortable.
- How to help someone learn daily tasks:
    - Break tasks into small steps (use pictures to show each step).
    - Practice together until they can do more by themselves.
    - Praise their effort and celebrate their progress.
    - Offer choices whenever possible (what to wear, what soap to use).
- Tools to help:
    - Picture cards (show each step in a routine).

- o Timers (show how long each step should take).
- Work with others:
  - o Family members should use the same techniques.
  - o Therapists can help with specific challenges.
  - o Teachers can help them practice at school too.
- Be patient and understanding, everyone learns at their own pace. By helping them learn daily tasks, they gain more confidence and independence.

Money management: Teaching financial responsibility

- Managing money is important for people with ID because it helps them:
  - o Be more independent (do things on their own).
  - o Avoid scams (make good choices about spending).
  - o Save for things they want (plan for the future).
- Learning about money can be hard because:
  - o Numbers and concepts can be confusing.
  - o Planning for the future is difficult.
  - o It is tempting to spend money right away.
- How to help someone learn about money:

- o Start with basics (teach about coins, bills, and their value).
- o Explain needs vs. wants (need food, want new toys).
- o Explain working and spending (earn money to spend wisely).
- Budgeting tips:
  - o Use pictures or apps to make it easier.
  - o Start simple (focus on few things like food).
  - o Practice with play money or apps.
- Good money habits:
  - o Track income (allowance, wages) and expenses (groceries, movies).
  - o Set spending limits for different things.
  - o Save for things they really want in the future.
- Overcoming challenges:
  - o Help them develop strategies to resist spending right away (wait a day to think).
  - o Provide extra help with apps if needed.
  - o Be patient, everyone learns at their own pace.
- Putting it into practice:
  - o Take them shopping (teach smart choices).
  - o Act out situations and practice good spending habits.
  - o Praise them for making good choices with money.

- Work with others:
  - o Family uses the same techniques to teach about money.
  - o Financial experts can help with complex situations.
  - o Job coaches can also help teach about money.
- Learning about money takes time and practice. By being patient and working together, you can help them feel more confident and in control of their money.

Cooking and meal preparation: Promoting healthy eating habits.

- Cooking is great for people with ID because it helps them:
  - o Eat healthy (choose ingredients and control portions).
  - o Be independent (cook their own meals).
  - o Feel good (build confidence by learning a new skill).
  - o Have fun with others (cooking can be a social activity).
- Learning to cook can be hard because:
  - o Using tools (knives, pots) can be difficult.
  - o Following steps in recipes can be confusing.

- o Kitchen sounds, smells, or textures might be overwhelming.
- Tips for safe and easy cooking:
  - o Start with simple recipes with few ingredients (use pictures for steps).
  - o Use timers and checklists to keep track.
  - o Use special tools like easy-grip knives or measuring cups.
- Learn to cook step-by-step:
  - o Cook together and let the person with ID help as much as possible.
  - o Teach safety rules (knives, hot things).
  - o Break down recipes into small steps and focus on one step at a time.
  - o Praise them for trying even if it is messy.
- Eating healthy foods while cooking:
  - o Use healthy ingredients like fruits, vegetables, and whole grains.
  - o Aim for balanced meals with protein, carbs, and healthy fats.
  - o Plan meals together and teach about healthy options.
  - o Make it fun with food group games or a healthy recipe book.
- Work with others:
  - o Cook healthy meals together as a family.
  - o Therapists can help with using hands and textures.

- o Nutritionists can help plan healthy meals and understand food labels.
- Learning to cook takes time and practice. Be patient and work together to help the person with ID cook healthy meals and have fun in the kitchen.

Transportation and mobility: Encouraging independent travel

- Benefits:
    - o Do more (go to work, school, visit others).
    - o Feel more grown-up (independent and confident).
    - o Learn new things (skills, explore the city).
- Challenges:
    - o Maps and schedules are confusing.
    - o Following steps is difficult.
    - o Crowds and noise can be overwhelming.
- Learning to travel safely:
    - o Teach street smarts (crossing streets, bike safety).
    - o Plan the trip together (familiar route, practice with pictures/maps).
    - o Practice social skills (talking to bus/train staff).
- Taking public transport alone:
    - o Start with short trips, gradually go further.
    - o Practice what to do if lost or miss a bus.
    - o Celebrate successful independent trips.

- Working together:
  - Family: Gradually let the person travel alone after practicing together.
  - Public transport: Ask how they can help people with ID travel safely.
  - Teachers/Therapists: Teach map reading, schedules, getting used to crowds/noise.
- Staying safe:
  - Teach how to find help if lost (police, asking for directions).
  - Discuss safety in unfamiliar areas (maybe travel with a friend at first).
  - Consider special safety tools (alarms, tracking devices).

Remember: Be patient, practice together, and celebrate successes. Traveling is a great way to learn and explore.

Time management skills: Developing routines and using tools like calendars and schedules

- Benefits:
  - Be more independent (do things on their own).
  - Feel less stressed and overwhelmed (know what to do next).
  - Get things done and reach goals (focus on important tasks).

- o Stay organized (appointments, on top of things).
- Challenges:
  - o Understanding time can be tricky.
  - o Remembering schedules and deadlines can be hard.
  - o Staying focused can be difficult.
- Making a daily plan:
  - o Use pictures and charts to show what to do and when.
  - o Try to keep a consistent routine (waking up, eating, sleeping).
  - o Break big tasks into smaller steps.
- Time management tools:
  - o Calendars or planner apps for appointments and reminders.
  - o Timers and alarms to switch activities and stay on schedule.
  - o Special apps with pictures for easy use.
- Getting better at time management:
  - o Practice using a schedule and tools regularly.
  - o Celebrate successes with using the tools.
  - o Start simple and gradually add more to the routine.
  - o Minimize distractions (headphones, quiet place to work).
- Feeling in control:

- o Help the person with ID decide what goes on their schedule.
  - o Offer choices within the routine and allow some flexibility.
  - o Celebrate the effort, even if things aren't perfect on time.
- Working together:
  - o Family members practice using a schedule with the person with ID.
  - o Therapists can help with focus strategies.
  - o Teachers can help teach time management skills at school.

Remember: Be patient, practice together, and celebrate successes. This will help them feel less stressed and achieve their goals.

Problem-solving skills: Encouraging critical thinking and independent decision-making.

- Benefits:
  - o Be more independent (solve problems by themselves).
  - o Learn from mistakes (try again after solving problems).
  - o Get along with others (work through disagreements).
  - o Get a job (problem-solving skills are important for many jobs).

- Challenges:
    - o Thinking about what might happen can be difficult.
    - o Making a plan to solve a problem can be hard.
    - o Waiting for the best answer can be difficult.
- Having a growth mindset:
    - o Everyone can learn from mistakes.
    - o Effort matters more than getting the right answer right away.
    - o See problems as challenges, not something to get upset about.
- Becoming a problem-solving star:
    - o Act out situations and practice solving problems together.
    - o Think of many solutions, even silly ones at first.
    - o Use pictures and charts to show problem-solving steps.
    - o Use special apps and tools to help think through problems.
- Making decisions on your own:
    - o Give small choices throughout the day to practice decision-making.
    - o Help with decisions at first, then gradually give more control.
    - o Celebrate trying to solve problems, even if the decision is not perfect.
- Working together:

- o Talk about problems and how to solve them as a family.
- o Therapists can help with communication during problem-solving.
- o Teachers can help practice problem-solving skills at school.

Remember: Be patient, practice together, and celebrate successes. This will help them feel more independent and in control.

Safety awareness

- Benefits of learning safety:
    - o Do more things independently (go more places).
    - o Avoid accidents and stay safe.
    - o Feel more confident and less scared.
    - o Interact with others safely.
- Challenges of learning safety:
    - o Understanding dangers can be difficult.
    - o Talking about safety can be hard.
    - o Loud noises or alarms can be overwhelming.
- Learning safety skills:
    - o Use simple words and short sentences.
    - o Show pictures and videos to explain safety rules.

- o Practice safety skills together (fire drills, meeting strangers).
- Fire safety:
  - o Learn escape plans for home, school, etc.
  - o Know what fire alarms sound like and what to do.
  - o Practice crawling low under smoke and getting out safely.
- Stranger danger:
  - o Learn who is safe to talk to and who to be careful around.
  - o Use the buddy system, especially in unfamiliar places.
  - o It is okay to say "no" and ask for help if you feel unsafe.
- Other safety skills:
  - o Learn street safety (crossing streets, riding a bike safely).
  - o Learn about personal safety (not sharing personal information, body safety, internet safety).
  - o Learn how to identify emergency personnel and call for help.

Remember: Be patient, practice together. This will help them feel more confident and independent.

Working together

- Practice safety skills and talk about safety rules as a family.
- Teachers can teach safety in school, therapists can help with communication or sensory issues.
- Some community programs can teach safety skills in a fun way.

Leisure and recreation

- Benefits of fun activities:
    - Feel better (reduce stress, feel happy).
    - Learn new things (from trying new activities).
    - Make friends (join group activities).
- Challenges of finding fun activities:
    - Maybe they have not tried many things.
    - Some activities might be too difficult.
    - Being around new people can be scary.
- Finding the perfect activity:
    - Talk about what they enjoy.
    - Explore places like museums or parks to see their interest.
    - Try different activities to see what is fun.
- Making activities accessible:
    - Use special tools (bigger paint brushes, balls with handles).

- o Help with social skills or find a buddy for the activity.
  - o Provide extra support if needed.
- Keeping the fun going:
  - o Focus on having fun, not being the best.
  - o Encourage them to try activities independently as they get better.
  - o Keep exploring to find new hobbies and interests.
- Working together:
  - o Families can try new activities together and encourage exploration.
  - o Teachers can teach leisure skills and therapists can help with social skills or limitations.
  - o Community programs offer activities designed for people with ID.

Remember: Be patient, explore together, and help them discover activities they love. Fun is important for everyone.

10. SOCIAL BUTTERFLIES

Understanding social cues and body language

- Benefits of understanding body language:
    - Know what others feel (happy, sad, mad, scared).
    - Make better friends and have stronger relationships.
    - Avoid misunderstandings and confusion.
    - Feel more confident talking to others.
- Challenges of understanding body language:
    - Faces and gestures can be confusing.
    - Less practice talking to others makes it harder to understand.
    - We focus too much on words and forget body language is important too.
- Learning the body language code:
    - Start with basics (happy, sad, mad, scared faces) using pictures and mirrors.
    - Act out situations and guess feelings based on body language.
    - Play matching games or watch videos about body language.
    - Learn body position (interested, bored, uncomfortable).
    - Learn about eye contact and personal space.
- Making it stick:

- o Practice regularly to improve understanding.
  - o Celebrate successes and effort in understanding body language.
  - o Participate in social activities to practice these skills.
- Working together:
  - o Family can talk about body language and practice at home.
  - o Teachers can teach body language in school; therapists can help with social anxiety or sensory issues.
  - o Social groups can help practice social skills and body language with peers.

Remember: Be patient, practice together. This will help them feel more confident and have stronger relationships. Body language is a big part of communication.

Building friendships

- Benefits of friends:
  - o Learn from each other (kindness, taking turns, feelings).
  - o Feel good and confident.
  - o Not feel alone.
  - o Do more fun things together.
- Challenges of making friends:

- o Talking can be tricky.
- o Feeling shy can be tough.
- o Finding friends with similar interests can be hard.
- Learning how to make friends:
  - o Practice social skills (greeting, taking turns, asking questions).
  - o Know your feelings and how to talk about them with friends.
  - o Respect personal space.
- Making friends happen:
  - o Join a club or group activity for things you like.
  - o Work together on school projects or play games with classmates.
  - o Play games that teach friendship skills.
- Keeping friendships strong:
  - o Learn how to play together (taking turns, sharing, listening).
  - o Be a good listener and show you care.
  - o Work through problems by talking and finding solutions together.
- Working together:
  - o Family can help set up playdates and practice social skills at home.
  - o Teachers can teach social skills in school, therapists can help with shyness or communication.

- o Community groups offer activities to meet new people and make friends.

Remember: Be patient, practice together. Friends make life more fun; everyone deserves good friends.

Dealing with bullying and social exclusion

- Bullies are mean people who can:
    - o Say mean things (name calling, making fun).
    - o Try to scare you (pushing, taking things).
    - o Leave you out of games.
- It can be hard for people with ID to know if someone is bullying because:
    - o They might not understand what is happening.
    - o They might be scared to tell someone.
- How to stay safe from bullies:
    - o Know the signs (name calling, pushing, taking things, leaving you out).
    - o Say no to bullies in a firm voice.
    - o Walk away and find a trusted grown-up for help.
- Make a plan to stay safe:
    - o Talk to a trusted grown-up about bullies.
    - o Practice what to say to a bully and how to ask for help.

- o Remember you are not alone; people care and want to help.
- Working together to stay safe:
  - o Family can talk about bullying and practice safety strategies.
  - o Teachers can teach about bullying and kindness. Therapists can help with anxiety or social skills.
  - o Schools can have anti-bullying rules to keep everyone safe.

Remember: Bullies are not nice but you can stay safe. By knowing the signs, having a plan, and working with others, you can feel safe and happy.

Promoting social inclusion

- Benefits of being involved:
  - o Make new friends with similar interests.
  - o Learn new things (sports, art classes, etc.).
  - o Feel good and confident.
  - o Practice independence, communication, and social skills.
- Challenges of getting involved:
  - o Finding activities that are inclusive (welcome everyone).
  - o Transportation challenges (no car, inaccessible public transport).
  - o Feeling scared about new places and people.

- o Let us make it happen.
- o Find activities they enjoy (talk to them and look for matching programs).
- o Ask around for inclusive programs (teachers, therapists, community centers).
- o Start small with short outings with support, then increase independence gradually.
- Helping your child shine:
  - o Practice social skills (greeting, taking turns, joining conversations).
  - o Celebrate their efforts and achievements, no matter how small.
  - o Be their buddy at first for support and to model behavior.
- Working together:
  - o Family: Help them find activities, practice skills, and celebrate successes.
  - o Teachers & Therapists: Organize community outings, teach social skills, address challenges.
  - o Community Programs: Create inclusive programs and accessible spaces.

Remember: Getting involved takes time and effort, but it is worth it. With planning and collaboration, you can help your child build a fulfilling life in the community. Everyone deserves to belong.

11. SELF-CARE FOR THE JOURNEY

Prioritizing your own mental and physical well-being

- Parents of children with ID need to take care of themselves too.
- Feeling stressed and tired makes it hard to be patient and have fun with your child.
- If you do not take care of yourself, you have less energy and love to give to your child.
- Taking care of yourself shows your child it is important to be healthy and happy.
- Do things you enjoy, even for a little while each day.
- Ask family, friends, or professionals for help.
- Join a support group to talk to other parents who understand.
- Eat healthy, sleep well, and exercise regularly.
- Talk to family and friends about the kind of help you need.
- Look for community resources like support groups or counseling.
- Do not be afraid to ask a therapist for help with stress or anxiety.
- Taking care of yourself is NOT selfish, it makes you a stronger parent

Finding support groups and connecting with other families

- Feeling alone raising a child with ID? You are not. There are many families out there who understand.
- Sharing your journey with others can help:
    o Find support and advice from parents who get it.
    o Learn new strategies and resources.
    o Feel hopeful and empowered by others' success.
- Find your support village:
    o Ask your doctor or child's school about local groups.
    o Search online for forums or social media groups for parents of children with ID.
- There are different types of support groups:
    o In-person groups for strong connections and community.
    o Online groups for flexibility if you are busy.
    o Specialized groups for specific needs.
- Get the most out of your support group:
    o Be open and share your experiences.
    o Offer support and encouragement to others.
    o Build lasting friendships.
- Do not forget to build a wider support system:

- o Consider therapy to manage stress or anxiety.
- o Explore respite care to take breaks and recharge.
- o Look into mentorship programs for guidance from experienced parents.

Remember, reaching out for support is a sign of strength. It helps you create a brighter future for your child. So, take that first step today.

Strategies for managing stress and avoiding burnout

- Raising a child with ID is amazing but stressful. Taking care of yourself is important.
- Stress makes it hard to be patient and can even make you sick.
- Find healthy ways to relax like reading, walking, or listening to music.
- It is okay to say no to extra things when you are overwhelmed.
- Talk to someone about how you are feeling - a therapist, counselor, or another parent.
- Do not be afraid to ask for help from family, friends, or professionals.
- Look into respite care to give yourself a break.
- Focus on the positive things in your life, big and small.

- Celebrate your victories, no matter how small.
- Remember why you love and care for your child.
- You are not alone. There are many parents who understand what you are going through.

Maintaining healthy relationships

- Raising a child with ID can be busy, but strong relationships are important.
- A good support system helps you manage stress and feel less alone.
- It gives you a break and allows you to be a better parent.
- It also helps your child feel loved and supported.
- Balancing relationships can be hard because:
  - There is not enough time.
  - People might not understand your challenges.
  - You might be too tired to talk.
- Here is how to keep your relationships strong:
  - Talk to your partner about your needs and share the parenting load.
  - Schedule date nights or outings, even if short.
  - Catch up with friends quickly over coffee or phone calls.
  - Include family in activities you enjoy.
  - Be realistic - quality over quantity.

- o Talk to friends and family about ID so they can understand.
- Connect with other parents who understand.
- Look into respite care to give yourself and your partner a break.
- Do not be afraid to ask for help with errands or childcare.
- Strong relationships are like a lifeline for you and your family.

Prioritizing relaxation and stress-reduction techniques

- Raising a child with ID is amazing but stressful. Taking care of yourself is important.
- Stress makes it hard to be a good parent and can even make you sick.
- Relaxation techniques can help you de-stress and feel better.
- Here are some relaxation techniques:
  - o Mindfulness and meditation: helps you focus on the present moment. There are apps to help you get started.
  - o Progressive muscle relaxation: tense and relax different muscle groups to release tension.
  - o Guided imagery: imagine yourself in a peaceful place to feel serene.
- Exercise is another great stress reliever:

- o Releases endorphins, which improve mood and reduce stress.
  - o Helps you sleep better.
  - o Improves focus and brain function.
  - o Reduces risk of health problems.
- Find hobbies you enjoy:
  - o Helps you relax and de-stress.
  - o Reminds you of who you are outside of caregiving.
  - o Connects you with others and fosters a sense of belonging.
  - o Offers a healthy outlet for emotions and can boost your mood.
- Tips for making relaxation a habit:
  - o Start small and gradually increase the time you spend relaxing.
  - o Try different techniques and hobbies to find what works for you.
  - o Schedule relaxation time in your day like any other appointment.
  - o Tell your partner or friends about your relaxation goals and ask for their support.
- Relaxation is self-care, not a luxury. There are many resources available to help you relax.

Respite care services

- Raising a child with special needs is rewarding, but tiring.
- Respite care gives parents a break from caregiving.
- Benefits of respite care:
    - Less stress and more patience for parents.
    - Stronger relationships with family and friends.
    - Time for parents to do things they enjoy.
- Types of respite care:
    - In-home care: Someone comes to your house.
    - Out-of-home care: Child stays in a safe place for short visits.
    - Family/friend care: A trusted person cares for your child temporarily.
    - Camp programs: Camps offer activities and socialization for children.
- Finding respite care:
    - Talk to your doctor for recommendations.
    - Contact local disability groups for info and financial assistance.
    - Search online for providers.
    - Talk to your child about respite care (if possible).
- Challenges:
    - Cost (financial assistance may be available).

- o Separation anxiety (open communication can help).
  - o Finding the right fit (explore different options).
- Respite care is not a sign of weakness, it helps parents be stronger caregivers.

Seeking professional help

- **Feeling Down?** Raising a child with ID can be stressful and make you feel anxious, depressed, or overwhelmed.
- **Take Care of Yourself.** Therapy can help you manage stress, improve communication with your child, and build a stronger support system.
- **It is Okay to Ask for Help.** Seeking therapy is a sign of strength, not weakness. There are therapists who specialize in helping parents like you.
- **Find the Right Fit:** Therapy comes in different forms like one-on-one sessions, couples therapy, or support groups. There are also options to make therapy affordable.

Maintaining a positive outlook

- **Focus on the good.** It helps you feel better and manage stress. It also strengthens the bond with your child.

- **Celebrate all victories, big or small.** Did your child learn a new word? Master a button closure? That is awesome.

- **Do not compare your child to others.** Every child learns at their own pace.

- **Keep track of your child's progress.** A journal or record helps you see how far they've come.

- **Celebrate together.** Make it a family affair and share your child's victories with friends and loved ones.

- **Celebrating victories helps your child too.** It boosts their confidence and makes them want to learn more.

- **Focus on the effort, not just the outcome.** Did your child try really hard to learn something new? That deserves a celebration.

12. BUILDING SIBLING BONDS

Fostering understanding and empathy among siblings

- Siblings of children with ID may feel confused, frustrated, isolated, or jealous.
- Fostering empathy helps siblings understand their sibling's needs, respond better to challenges, and offer support.
- Here is how to build empathy:
    - o Talk openly and honestly about your child with ID's disability.
    - o Explain that everyone is different with strengths and weaknesses.
    - o Schedule playtime and activities for siblings to connect.
    - o Act out situations to practice how to be empathetic.
    - o Praise siblings for being understanding, kind, and patient.
- Address jealousy by giving each child individual attention and acknowledging their feelings.
- Help your child with ID make friends outside the family.
- Consider professional help if siblings struggle a lot.
- Empathy leads to a stronger sibling bond, increased self-esteem, and a supportive family environment.

- Talk openly, address concerns, and create opportunities for connection to build a strong and lasting sibling bond.

Encouraging shared activities and creating opportunities for connection

- Families with a child with ID can benefit from shared activities:
    - Creates a stronger family bond.
    - Improves communication and understanding.
    - Builds memories and happiness.
- There are challenges to shared activities:
    - Finding accessible activities.
    - Limited time due to caregiving demands.
    - Activities might be frustrating for some.
- Here is how to overcome the challenges:
    - Plan adaptable activities for all abilities.
    - Focus on fun and be flexible.
    - Start with short activities and gradually increase the time.
    - Involve your child with ID in planning the activities.
- Examples of shared activities:
    - Adapted games, arts and crafts, outdoor activities, sensory play, family meals.
- Celebrate individuality:

- o Plan activities that cater to everyone's strengths and interests.
  - o Acknowledge everyone's effort and participation.
  - o Embrace your child with ID's unique needs and preferences.
- Benefits of connection:
  - o Reduces sibling resentment.
  - o Improves social skills for your child with ID.
  - o Increases confidence and self-esteem for everyone.
- Shared activities create a supportive family environment:
  - o Less isolation and resentment among siblings.
  - o Stronger family bond and joyful memories.
- Celebrate your unique strengths as a family.

Addressing sibling rivalry and jealousy

- Siblings of a child with ID may feel jealous and upset because they get less attention or do not understand their sibling's needs.
- Here is how to address sibling rivalry and jealousy:
  - o Talk openly and honestly about feelings, and let them know it is okay to feel jealous.
  - o Explain their sibling's disability and why they need extra help.

- o Listen to their concerns and comfort them.
- o Praise siblings for being kind, patient, and helpful to their sibling with ID.
- o Spend quality time with each child one-on-one.
- o Involve siblings in helping care for their sibling with ID (age-appropriate tasks).
- o Help siblings understand their sibling's perspective through books, videos, or talks.
- o Act out situations to practice how to be patient and helpful.
- o Celebrate the times siblings get along and play together.
- By talking openly and rewarding good behavior, you can help siblings feel better and build a stronger bond.
- This creates a more supportive and inclusive family environment for everyone.

Celebrating the unique bond between siblings of a Child with ID

- Siblings of a child with ID share a special bond.
- They grow up together, understand each other well, and have a unique way of communicating.
- They may also face challenges like confusion, jealousy, or not knowing their role in the family.
- Here is how to celebrate the sibling bond:

- o Acknowledge that their relationship is special.
  - o Celebrate achievements of both children.
  - o Give siblings time to connect and play together.
  - o Encourage open communication about their feelings.
  - o Recognize acts of kindness, patience, and understanding between siblings.
- Celebrating this bond creates a strong and supportive family.
- Siblings feel good about themselves and their role in the family.
- They develop important social skills and become lifelong friends.
- The sibling bond is strong and deserves to be celebrated.

Addressing sibling guilt and resentment

- Siblings of a child with ID may feel guilt (not doing enough) and resentment (limitations, unmet needs)
- These feelings can hurt the sibling relationship and cause other problems.
- Here is how parents can help:
  - o Allow siblings to talk freely about their feelings without judgment.

- o Let them know it is okay to feel guilt and resentment.
  - o Explain these are normal emotions and there are healthy ways to deal with them.
  - o Clear up any misconceptions about their sibling's disability.
- Spend quality time with each child and acknowledge their efforts.
- Help siblings understand their sibling's perspective.
- Teach siblings healthy ways to cope with difficult emotions.
- Plan activities that everyone can enjoy together.
- Celebrate positive interactions between siblings.
- Consider support groups for siblings of children with ID.
- By talking openly and offering support, parents can help siblings deal with guilt and resentment in a healthy way.
- This leads to a stronger sibling bond, better self-esteem for everyone, and a more supportive family environment.

Encouraging sibling participation in caregiving

- Siblings can help care for their brother or sister with ID in age-appropriate ways.
- This helps everyone:
  - o Stronger sibling bond.
  - o More empathy and understanding.

- o Better communication skills.
- o Feels good for the sibling who helps.
- There can be challenges:
  - o Tasks must be the right difficulty level.
  - o Siblings may not want the extra work.
  - o There is not always a lot of time.
- Here is how to overcome the challenges:
  - o Start with small tasks and make them harder over time.
  - o Make helping fun and focus on working together.
  - o Talk about what needs to be done and listen to any problems.
  - o Praise siblings for their effort, even if they do not do everything perfectly.
- Examples of how siblings can help:
  - o Younger: Set the table, sort toys, play together.
  - o Teenager: Reminders for medicine, prepare snacks, light chores together.
  - o Older: Help with personal care (with guidance), talk together, go places together.
- Working together as a team helps everyone:
  - o Less stress for parents.
  - o Siblings learn responsibility and empathy.
  - o Siblings feel important to the family.
- By working together, siblings can build a strong and supportive family.

Celebrating sibling differences

- All siblings have different strengths: talents, personalities, communication styles, and problem-solving approaches.
- It is important to celebrate these strengths in each child, not just focus on the child with ID's challenges.
- Here is how to celebrate strengths:
  - Notice and praise each child's unique talents.
  - Encourage them to explore their interests and get better at what they like.
  - Focus on what each child can do well, not what they cannot do.
  - Plan activities that let each child show off their strengths.
- Celebrate how siblings work together using their strengths to help each other.
- Use positive language to talk about all the different strengths in the family.
- Each child brings something special to the family.
- By celebrating differences, siblings feel good about themselves, the bond gets stronger, and everyone learns to accept others who are different.
- Every child's voice matters in the family.

Building a lifelong support system

- Siblings of a child with ID can be lifelong friends and supporters for each other.
- This is important because siblings understand each other well and can be there for each other through life.
- There are challenges to staying close as siblings grow up, like distance and busy lives.
- Here is how to help siblings stay close:
    - Encourage positive interactions and open communication from a young age.
    - Plan activities and create memories together throughout their lives.
    - Help siblings use technology to stay connected if they live far apart.
    - Educate friends and partners about the sibling relationship and ID.
    - Respect each sibling's life choices and needs.
- By staying close, siblings can feel less stressed, have better social lives, and advocate for each other.
- A strong sibling bond is a gift that lasts a lifetime.

13. FINANCIAL PLANNING

Understanding financial resources available to families with ID

- Raising a child with ID can be expensive.
- There are resources to help, including:
    - Government programs like SSI, SSDI, Medicaid, and IDEA
    - Community support from disability rights organizations, vocational rehab, and charities
    - Tax benefits like the Dependent Care Tax Credit and Disability Tax Credit
- Getting these resources can be complicated because of eligibility requirements, limited funding, and lack of awareness.
- Here is how to get help:
    - Research programs and contact disability rights organizations or social service agencies.
    - Consider getting a lawyer to help with applications.
    - Be prepared to advocate for your child and be persistent.
- Financial planning is also important:
    - Think about long-term care needs as your child gets older.

- o Consider special needs trusts to protect benefits.
- o Save for your child's future using options like ABLE accounts.
- It takes effort to get financial help, but it can make a big difference for your child.

Government benefits and assistance programs

- Different countries offer different benefits, but some common ones are:
  - o Disability benefits (money to help with costs of care)
- Healthcare coverage (medical insurance)
  - o Education support (special needs teachers, therapists)
  - o Respite care (help for families to take a break)
- You need to research what your country offers specifically. Here is how to find out:
  - o Look at government websites
  - o Contact disability rights organizations
  - o Ask social service agencies
- Tips for applying for benefits:
  - o Collect documents about your child's disability
  - o Meet deadlines
  - o Appeal decisions if needed

- There is more help available beyond government benefits:
  - Community organizations (support groups, workshops)
  - Charities (financial assistance, donations)

Securing the Future

- Planning for your child's future finances is important because:
  - They may need ongoing support.
  - Inheritance could affect eligibility for government benefits.
- Financial planning can help:
  - Keep government benefits.
  - Ensure a good quality of life for your child.
  - Give you peace of mind.
- Special Needs Trusts (SNTs) are a legal tool to manage money for someone with a disability:
  - There are two types: set up with the disabled person's money or with someone else's money.
  - The money in the trust does not count against the disabled person for benefits.
  - The trustee can use the money for things not covered by benefits, like extra care or activities.
- Other financial planning tips:

- o Life insurance can provide money for your child after you die.
- o Some government programs let you save money for a disabled person (e.g. ABLE accounts in the US).
- o Talk to a financial advisor about investments.
- To get started:
  - o Talk to a lawyer about what type of SNT is best for you.
  - o Talk to a financial planner who works with families with disabled children.
  - o Discuss your plans with your child (if appropriate) and other family members.
- By planning for the future, you can make sure your child has the support they need throughout their life.

Utilizing insurance coverage effectively

- Health insurance can help pay for medical costs for your child with ID. There are 3 main types:
  - o Private insurance (work or individual plan)
  - o Government programs (Medicaid/PIP)
  - o Disability waivers (extra coverage within Medicaid)
- Make sure you understand what your plan covers by:
  - o Reading your plan documents

- o Calling your insurance company
  - o Talking to your child's doctor
- Here are some tips to get the most out of your insurance:
  - o Get pre-authorization before some treatments
  - o See in-network providers to save money
  - o Keep good records of your child's care
  - o Appeal denied claims if you have documentation
- Sometimes you may need to fight for coverage:
  - o Get a letter from your doctor explaining why the treatment is needed
  - o Request an independent medical review if your appeal is denied
  - o Contact disability rights organizations for help
- Other things to keep in mind:
  - o Some plans have lifetime maximums on benefits
  - o You may want to consider long-term care insurance
  - o Keep your doctor and insurance company informed of any changes
- By understanding your insurance and advocating for your child, you can make sure they get the care they need.

14. PLANNING FOR THE FUTURE

Guardianship options

- Guardianship is a legal arrangement where someone makes decisions for an adult who cannot make their own choices.
- This might be needed for your child with ID if they cannot manage their money, healthcare, or daily living.
- There are 2 types of guardianship:
    - Guardian of the Person: decides on where your child lives, their medical care, and well-being.
    - Guardian of the Estate: manages your child's money, property, and investments.
- Setting up guardianship involves courts and evaluations.
- Courts prefer to give people as much independence as possible before guardianship.
- Here is how to choose a guardian:
    - Someone who understands intellectual disabilities and your child's needs.
    - Someone who shares your values for your child's care.
    - Someone willing and able to handle the responsibility.
    - Someone you and your child trust to communicate openly.

- Alternatives to guardianship include:
  - Supported decision-making agreements: someone helps your child make decisions but they can still participate.
  - Durable powers of attorney: someone you trust can manage your child's finances or healthcare if they cannot.
- Planning for the future shows you love your child.
- The goal is to give your child the support they need while letting them be as independent as possible.

Transition to adulthood
:

- Helping your child with ID prepare for adulthood:
  - Find their strengths and interests for future jobs.
  - Consider vocational assessments and training programs.
  - Supported employment programs can provide job coaching.
  - Look for community-based training for practical skills.
- Teach your child life skills:
  - Taking care of themselves (hygiene, dressing)
  - Managing money
  - Cooking
  - Using public transportation

- Help them develop social skills:
    - o Encourage interaction with others and community activities.
    - o Teach them to speak up for themselves.
    - o Help them make decisions on their own.
- Explore independent living options:
    - o Supported living with some help nearby.
    - o Programs to teach them how to manage a home on their own.
    - o Talk to your child about what they want.
    - o Look for organizations that can help with independent living.
- Tips for success:
    - o Start planning early.
    - o See if there are government programs that can help.
    - o Talk to teachers, therapists and disability rights groups for advice.
    - o Keep talking to your child about their future and celebrate their achievements.

Long-term care planning

- Planning long-term care for your adult child with ID:
    - o Think about where they will live:
        - ▪ Family home (with maybe changes to make it safe and accessible)

- Supported living (independent living with help nearby)
        - Group homes (shared living with daily support)
        - Care homes (structured environment with 24/7 supervision)
    - Consider your child's needs, preferences, and budget when choosing a place.
- There are also support services to help your child:
    - Habilitation services (learn daily living skills)
    - Vocational support (job training and help finding a job)
    - Therapy services (speech, occupational, behavioral)
    - Social and recreational activities
    - Medical and dental care
- Talk to your child about their future and what they want.
- Think about how their needs might change and if their living situation can change too.
- Look into legal options like guardianship to make sure your child is always cared for.
- Build a strong support network of family and friends.
- This is an ongoing process, but by planning ahead you can help your child live a good life.

Addressing end-of-life decisions

- Talking about end-of-life care with your child with ID is hard, but important.
- If your child can understand, talk to them about it in a calm and private place.
- Start with general talks about death and dying using words they understand.
- Focus on what matters to your child, not the specifics of medical treatments.
- You may need to be their legal guardian to make healthcare choices.
- Advance directives can express your child's wishes for future care.
- Talk to a lawyer who specializes in disability law.
- Learn about hospice care, pain management, and palliative care.
- Discuss treatment options with your child's doctor.
- Quality of life is most important - avoid unnecessary suffering.
- Consider your child's cultural and religious beliefs.
- Include family members in discussions for support.
- Prepare for grief and loss after your child passes away.
- There are grief counseling and support groups available.
- Open communication and planning can help you make the best choices for your child.

15. CELEBRATING SUCCESS

Importance of recognizing achievements

- Celebrate your child with ID's achievements to boost their confidence.
- It can be anything big or small - every step counts.
- Why it matters:
    - Makes them feel good about themselves
    - Wants them to try harder next time
    - Makes your bond stronger
    - Teaches them that effort matters
- How to celebrate effectively:
    - Do what your child likes
    - Talk about how hard they worked
    - Tell them exactly what they did well
    - Make it fun with their favorite things
    - Include other people to celebrate with them
- Not just words. You can also:
    - Give them a small reward
    - Make a "success board" to show their achievements
    - Let them stay up a bit late or pick a bedtime story
    - Share their success with others with their permission
- Celebrate every step of the way:
    - Learned a new skill? Great.

- o Finished homework? Awesome.
- o Tried to make a friend? You did great.
- o Dealt with a problem? You are strong.
- Celebrating achievements is an investment in their future.
- It shows them you believe in them and helps them reach their dreams.

Creating traditions and rituals to acknowledge achievements

- Make traditions to celebrate your child with ID's achievements.
- Traditions are special ways to celebrate that you do again and again.
- They are good because:
  - o They make your child excited to achieve things.
  - o They show your child that their achievements are important.
  - o They make your family closer.
  - o They comfort your child with familiar routines.
- How to create traditions:
  - o Do something your child likes.
  - o Start small and add more as your child gets better at things.
  - o Make it fun with things they enjoy (food, music, activities).

- o Have different traditions for different size achievements (big vs small).
  - o Use traditions from your culture to celebrate.
- Here are some tradition ideas:
  - o Achievement Jar: Add something to the jar for each accomplishment, then empty it and celebrate together later.
  - o Success Menu: Choose a reward from a menu you make together after achieving a goal.
  - o Memory Wall: Show off their achievements, pictures, and art.
  - o Community Celebration: Have a party with friends or a support group (with your child's permission).
- Celebrate every step of the way.
  - o Learned a new skill? Have a movie night.
  - o Finished homework? Do a special handshake.
  - o Dealt with a problem? Go to the park.
- Traditions show your child you are proud of them and help them succeed.

Setting realistic goals and celebrating progress along the way

- Setting goals you can reach helps your child with ID succeed:

- o They feel good about themselves when they achieve something.
  - o They want to keep trying for new goals.
  - o They learn to do things on their own.
  - o They get less frustrated.
- How to set good goals:
  - o Pick things your child is good at and likes to do.
  - o Break big goals into small steps. Celebrate each step.
  - o Consider your child's individual needs and how they learn.
  - o Let your child help pick their goals (when possible).
  - o Ask therapists, teachers or other professionals for advice.
- Celebrate every step of the way, not just the finish line:
  - o Praise their effort, not just the final result.
  - o Tell them exactly what they did well.
  - o Celebrate in a way they like (favorite activity, small reward).
  - o Share their progress with family and friends.
  - o Make a chart to see their progress and celebrate completed steps.
- Be flexible:
  - o Goals may change as your child grows and learns.

- o Celebrate when they overcome challenges, even if they do not reach the final goal yet.
- o Focus on what they learn along the way, not just the end result.
- Setting goals and celebrating progress helps your child with ID be successful.

Finding joy in the journey

- Raising a child with ID is special. Here is why:
  - o They have unique talents you can celebrate (art, music, kindness).
  - o They learn in different ways, find what works for them.
  - o Every little improvement is a big win.
  - o They can make you see the beauty in simple things.
- Focus on the positive:
  - o See challenges as learning experiences for you and your child.
  - o Celebrate how your child overcomes obstacles.
  - o Enjoy learning new things alongside your child.
  - o Talk to other parents of children with ID for advice and support.
- Tips for finding joy:
  - o Take care of yourself so you can take care of your child.

- o Spend time with loved ones who support you.
- o Be proud of all you do for your child.
- Parenting a child with ID can be tough, but it is also rewarding.
- Focus on their strengths, enjoy the little things, and find joy in your unique relationship.

Building a legacy of love and acceptance

- Sharing your story about raising a child with ID can help others:
    - o People learn more about ID and understand it better.
    - o You connect with other parents who are going through the same thing.
    - o You give hope and advice to other parents.
    - o People become more accepting of people with ID.
- How to share your story:
    - o Think about what message you want to tell (love, acceptance, etc.).
    - o Write about it online, join a support group, or talk to a local newspaper.
    - o Be yourself and share your real experiences (both happy and hard).
    - o Focus on the positive things about your child and your life together.

- o Celebrate your child's achievements, big or small.
- You can also show love and acceptance by:
  - o Fighting for your child's rights in your community.
  - o Teaching others about ID in a nice way.
  - o Celebrating the things that make your child unique.
  - o Acting like everyone should accept people with ID.
- By sharing your story, you help create a world where everyone is accepted for who they are.
- Your story can inspire others and make the world a better place for people with ID.

Resources

List of some reputable websites focused on intellectual disability from various countries:

- **United States:** The Arc - [thearc.org]
  The Arc is a leading national organization advocating for and serving people with intellectual and developmental disabilities and their families.

- **United Kingdom**: Mencap [mencap.org.uk]
  Mencap is the UK's leading charity for people with a learning disability, providing support and promoting inclusion.

- **Canada:** Canadian Association for Community

Living (CACL) - [cacl.ca] CACL advocates for the rights and inclusion of people with intellectual disabilities across Canada.

- **Australia:** Inclusion Australia - [inclusionaustralia.org.au]
This organization focuses on the inclusion of people with intellectual disabilities in all aspects of community life.

- **Ireland:** Inclusion Ireland - [inclusionireland.ie]
Inclusion Ireland is the national association advocating for the rights of people with intellectual disabilities in Ireland.

- **New Zealand:** IHC New Zealand - [ihc.org.nz]
IHC New Zealand advocates for the rights, inclusion, and welfare of all people with intellectual disabilities.

- **India:** National Trust for the Welfare of Persons with Autism, Cerebral Palsy, Mental Retardation, and Multiple Disabilities - [thenationaltrust.gov.in]
This governmental organization focuses on promoting the well-being of persons with intellectual and developmental disabilities in India.

- **South Africa:** Down Syndrome South Africa (DSSA) - [downsyndromedssa.org.za]
DSSA is dedicated to improving the quality of life for individuals with Down syndrome and other intellectual disabilities.

- **Japan:** Japanese Society for Rehabilitation of Persons with Disabilities (JSRPD) - [dinf.ne.jp] JSRPD provides resources and support for people with disabilities, including intellectual disabilities, in Japan.

- **Sweden:** Swedish National Association for Persons with Intellectual Disability (FUB) - [fub.se] FUB works for better living conditions and opportunities for people with intellectual disabilities in Sweden.

- **Singapore:** MINDS (Movement for the Intellectually Disabled of Singapore) - [minds.org.sg] MINDS is one of Singapore's oldest and largest social service agencies, dedicated to providing comprehensive services for individuals with intellectual disabilities. They offer education, employment, and residential care services, among others.

These websites offer resources, support, and advocacy for individuals with intellectual disabilities and their families in their respective countries.

ABOUT THE AUTHOR

Dr. A. Mitra is a retired medical doctor who has worked in the field of General Practice in Family Medicine in India and Australia for over 30 years. He completed his graduate education in India and then did further studies in Australia and UK. Currently he lives a private modest life and pursues his interests in reading and writing on various topics.